## REAL wellness
It's what's new in wellness today

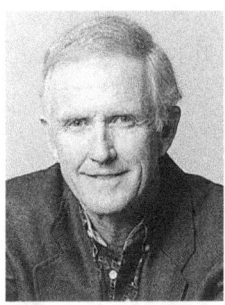

Donald B. Ardell publishes the ARDELL WELLNESS REPORT, a global newsletter on REAL™ wellness. Over 600 editions have been distributed worldwide since 1984. Dr. Ardell wrote the landmark best seller *High Level Wellness, an Alternative to Doctors, Drugs and Disease* in 1977 and over a dozen books since, including *The Book of Wellness: A Secular Approach to Spirituality, Meaning and Purpose, Die Healthy* and *Aging Beyond Belief*. Find him on the web at seekwellness.com. He is a board member of the United Nations Association in his area and trustee of the National Wellness Association. Don speaks regularly to audiences in Australia, Japan, Germany and other countries throughout the world. He is a world champion triathlete, twenty times all-American and member of the US Team. Recent successes include a world championship in 2009 (Gold Coast, Australia) and previously in Montreal and Hobart.

## Contents

## 1. Introduction: a message from the author

Wellness is a lifestyle founded on personal responsibility for your own well-being. I encourage you to discuss the tips and principles described in this book with your family, friends and associates.

Your well-being is the primary concern. By reading and discussing the concepts described here and exploring other REAL wellness ideas, you will continue to advance your lifestyle. This pleases me, for I want you to sustain the positive feelings and perspectives from this book long after your reading.

A Taoist saying, "The journey is the reward," captures the intention that wellness skills and practices are best implemented over time, little by little and bit by bit. What you do over the long haul is the truest measure, not the short bursts of temporary enthusiasms. There is no deadline, no rush for shaping a healthy, happy life. My own preference to proceeding with healthy lifestyle changes is to do so in a deliberate, sustainable pace, adding positive practices gradually, with time allotted for awareness, adjustments and ample reinforcements. To travel hopefully, at a leisurely pace, is better than to speed toward arrival or, as Robert Louis Stevenson gracefully wrote in *Virginibus Puerisque* (1881), "Little do ye know your own blessedness; for to travel hopefully is a better thing than to arrive, and the true success is to labour."

I hope you find this book a special gift. It is for you, with complements.

Welcome and enjoy.

## 2. Health, wellness and REAL wellness

Health is a term we associate with not being ill. That is the way most people understand being healthy. It is a very good thing not to be ill. However, we know there is a level of functioning that offers a higher level of health than simply not being ill. The World Health Organization has often made this point. Many people interested in exceptional health have, for at least half a century, given a special name to a lifestyle envisioned for high levels of health and well-being. That name is "wellness." I have promoted wellness since the early 1970's—my first book, a best seller, was called *High Level Wellness: an Alternative to Doctors, Drugs and Disease.* The emphasis in the wellness movement has been on personal responsibility, exercise and fitness, nutrition, stress management and environmental sensitivity.

Recently, a new term for advanced health has come into existence. It is called REAL wellness. That is the concept employed in this book. It includes the original ideas associated with wellness, but emphasizes the mental dimension as well as the physical. It describes a dynamic and comprehensive form of healthy living, at all stages of life, in sickness as well as in health.

REAL wellness is a positive approach to living designed to enhance quality of life. It is positive in that the motivation for making choices is well-being for its own sake, not avoiding weight gain, lowering risks of illness or extending longevity. It entails an active pursuit of vigorous exercise and fitness, sound nutrition, stress management and positive perspectives. But these are just for starters!

REAL wellness is not a product, a healing remedy or a medical service. It's not something someone else (e.g., a chiropractor or medical doctor), a clinic, spa or fitness center can deliver or administer. REAL wellness is an approach to the way you choose to think and act.

REAL is a modifier for the term wellness. It's an attempt to rescue the term from a great deal of woeful misuse. REAL wellness is an acronym that highlights four vital wellness qualities usually neglected, even ignored entirely, by those who use the word to promote a product, a healing remedy, a medical service or some other distracting misuse of the word.

REAL stands for nothing less than reason, exuberance, athleticism and liberty. It has four distinct qualities:

1. It is evidence-based (reason), rational and consistent with science—not testimonials or anecdotes of effectiveness.

2. It encourages joy, pleasure, fun and delight—not coping.

3. It promotes and entails maximum choice, freedom and liberty—not rules or restrictions.

4. It focuses on advances in quality of life—not risk reduction, illness management or life extension.

Based on increasing levels of desirability and significance, five kinds of wellness can be identified.

- Wellness as pampering and pleasure. That's spa wellness.
- Wellness as healing and rehabilitation. That's medical wellness.
- Wellness as a weight loss program. That's problem amelioration wellness.
- Wellness as fitness testing and prescriptions. That's risk reduction wellness.

- Wellness as explorations of reason, exuberant living and expanding personal freedoms, all in the service of increasing quality of life. That's REAL wellness.

A few leading questions:

Be brutally honest—is it realistic to expect wellness programs to convey more than risk reduction information? Can you comfortably evaluate pathways for personal responsibility, exercise and fitness, nutrition, stress and disease management? How about advancing the art and science of critical thinking along with exuberance, joy and pleasure? Other elements that fit with this mindset are sound relationships, emotional intelligence, happiness, resilience, ways to be a better global citizen, and the experience of being alive. (See my daily DBRU recommendation in the REAL wellness supplement at the end of the book.)

If you consider such an agenda attractive, and I suspect you do, REAL wellness will be a welcome part of your philosophy for living well.

Consider this simple graphic. It shows a continuum of health status from death/illness across an imaginary divide to REAL wellness.

## Continuum from Prevention to REAL wellness

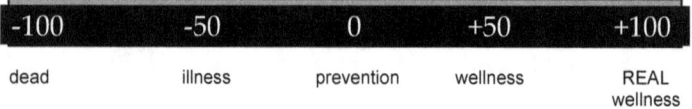

| -100 | -50 | 0 | +50 | +100 |
|------|-----|---|-----|------|
| dead | illness | prevention | wellness | REAL wellness |

Inasmuch as most people are overweight, unfit and fond of numerous dreadful habits that diminish health status, it's safe to conclude that most lifestyles tend to cluster on the left side of the continuum. Health educators spend most of their energy dealing with problems of sickness, risks and preventing things from getting worse.

| prevention | wellness | REAL wellness |
|------------|----------|---------------|
| risk assessment questionnaire | fitness and exercise | meaning and purpose |
| a medical self-care book | nutrition | positive psychology (understanding happiness) |
| weight loss/smoking clinics | stress management | fit, fun, free, functional |
| risk factors | building social support | critical thinking |
| medical management | environmental information | applied ethics |

Prevention, traditional health education—which constitutes the menu at most worksite wellness programs—has limited appeal. It is time to transition from medically-focused, left-brain warnings about the dangers of not choosing healthy lifestyles. Toward what, you ask? Toward right-brain feeling state connections between choices made daily and positive qualities available now. Including bust-your-buns exercise, or at least going for a good walk twice a day or the equivalent.

Maybe we should focus less on good health and more on a good life with a fit body. The good life, of course, starts with exceptional fitness—vigorous daily exercise, every day (alright, a day off now and then). REAL wellness promoters are not the first to carry on in this fashion. I suspect REAL wellness messages boosted Aristotle's career as a best-selling Greek philosopher and media star of his day (384 BCE - 322 BCE). That's what got him out from under the wing of his domineering tutor, Professor Plato. Aristotle's message to *his* prize pupil, Alexander the Great, was that "eudaimonia" (Greek, meaning happiness, human flourishing) and personal development to the fullest, ensues from vigorous daily exercise and service to others. Aristotle said little or nothing about not smoking, carousing, drinking too much, avoiding sloth or prevention.

Wellness is not a state of being but a process or style of living. The eminent psychologist Carl Rogers said as much when he described a good life. He called a good life, wellness to us, a direction, not a destination.

Of course, a feeling state for the experience of REAL wellness needs a proper context. We are not islands, as John Donne (1572-1631) noted. We're all pieces of the continent, parts of the main, involved in mankind. Try to go it alone with heroic individual efforts and bells may well toll for thee. Highly fit people need supportive, inspirational communities to get and stay that way. These might be family-based, sub-culture groups, associations and/or REAL wellness-oriented worksites with favorable life-supportive standards and customs.

In such REAL wellness environments, people know that regular vigorous exercise is expected; they feel they belong, they care about those around them and they feel respected and engaged in activities of value.

Which, of course, are all elements on the right side of the continuum, REAL wellness ingredients for positive living—not prevention. Now you know the differences between prevention and REAL wellness.

## 3. A REAL wellness personal plan

This book can be helpful if you wish to sketch a personal REAL wellness plan. Such a plan will help you make the most of opportunities to make healthy choices if and when you are not surrounded by the most positive or supportive culture.

It is sometimes said, or written in famous books, that these are the best of times, or the worst of times. A good case can always be made for one of these two extremes, or something in between.

My advice is don't concern yourself even for a moment with such matters. It does not matter. What difference does it make if Dickens thought things were tough during the French Revolution, or during the Stone Age, the Copper Age, the Bronze Age, the Iron Age or the Age of Aquarius? Who cares? This is *your* Age. This book will give you ideas for making the most of your time—here and now. This is the time to live in a manner that supports your best chances for happiness, health, meaning, exuberance and a life of reason with plenty of love given and received. These are quality of life areas you shape day after day.

So, in your hands, at this time, rests the chance to shape a small part of the world—the part you inhabit, for good or not. A REAL wellness lifestyle is something you deserve! Decide that you owe it to yourself to live well and you owe it, as well, to your family, your community and last, but not least, to your country. Get patriotic about it and choose a REAL wellness based lifestyle.

The limited role of medical ministrations:

REAL wellness is a commitment to behaviors, throughout each day, that boost quality of life. No medical system can ever do that, no matter how efficient. Medical resources are devoted to repairs— and the goals under the best of circumstances are actions to recover from illness and injury and advice designed to avoid breakdowns. Modern medicine's a wonderful thing but there are two problems: People expect too much of it and too little of themselves. This is not true for those who embrace REAL wellness.

REAL wellness is not reactive (i.e., designed to fix breakdowns); it is positive (i.e., designed to advance a better degree of functioning). REAL wellness is a mindset wherein you see yourself as the key variable, the accountable agent who alone can make life as agreeable as possible. REAL wellness entails attention to the experience of being alive, to happiness, to reasoned decision-making, to environmental awareness and to ethical choices. The latter is even more important in the new global order wherein many top business leaders, politicians and institutional representatives have distorted, squandered, plundered and manipulated public trust. What's required is a new era of responsibility and exuberant well-being.

The economy—important but not more than all else:

If unemployed or underemployed, suffering from a stock market that has tanked or hurt by failing business due to a credit crisis and arrested consumer spending, then the economy is major. Recently, our nation's leader said, "The state of our economy is a concern that rises above all others." While true in one sense, your first concern must be the state of your own life pattern. This state, the quality of your life, is affected by but not entirely dependent upon the economy. If your body is falling apart, this should be "a concern that rises above all others." Translation: Your lifestyle must be priority number one, always, in good times, bad times or any other kind of times!

Of course, this is not an either/or choice: a personal commitment to live well can be a fine companion to the national agendas of leaders seeking to renew a nation's promise. What you do to boost the quality of your life will matter most.

Doubt and skepticism are recommended elements of REAL wellness. This means always being willing to ask, "How do you know?" and insisting on credible, verifiable source data. To value liberty means being free from superstitions (e.g., good luck charms, fortune tellers, astrology) and arbitrary rules common to cults with their limitations based on dogma and archaic, irrational rules. As Harry Browne defined it, freedom means living your life as you see fit, pursuing whatever purpose you choose for yourself.

We are, of course, subject to the same limitations that protect the rights of all. Be sure to grant others freedoms that you desire. We all want equal rights in order to set our own course.

Speaking about freedom, the great 19th century orator Robert Ingersoll believed that freedom depended upon a citizenry that valued reason over superstition, respect for science over blind faith. He saw reason as a quality under assault from authoritarians—and urged us to protest it: "I admit that reason is a small and feeble flame, a flickering torch by stumblers carried in the starless night—blown and flared by passion's storm—and yet, it is the only light. Extinguish that, and nought remains." Ingersoll, who lived from 1833 to 1899, is considered a wellness pioneer as well as a great defender of reason, science and freedom.

Take little steps to gain added freedoms. For example—even something as modest as deciding to care a bit less about others approval will be beneficial. Liberty—which Ingersoll considered "the blossom and fruit of justice, the perfume of mercy"—is as important as daily exercise in the life-long enjoyment of a REAL wellness lifestyle. Woody Allen once cracked, "More than any time in history mankind faces a crossroads. One path leads to despair and utter hopelessness, the other to total extinction. Let us pray that we have the wisdom to choose correctly." Is it really that bad, or are there other paths, some more hopeful?

The whole point of wellness is quality of life. You know if you are enjoying it or not. You do not need to be tested, monitored, lectured, pressured, coached and/or mentored incessantly to reduce self-destructive behaviors. With a wellness mindset, you do the right thing because *you* value the outcomes.

REAL wellness might not be within everyone's reach. You are best positioned to assess your own chances. Throughout Europe and around the world, worksites are at something of a crossroads along lines that Woody Allen mentioned. Companies want to reduce worker morbidity and mortality. But, they overlooked a path that leads to quality of life enhancements for their employees. This is the REAL (reason, exuberance, athleticism and liberty) wellness road. This road has the valued side effect of reducing morbidity and mortality, even though that is not the prime focus for REAL wellness.

Studies support the belief that the highest returns for institutions that invest in wellness derive from quality of life choices, not prevention strategies. The report, "Health and productivity as a business strategy" in the Journal of Occupational and Environmental Medicine (Volume 49, # 7, July 2007) evaluated health-related lost productivity caused by medical conditions (including drug costs). The key findings were: 1) health-related productivity costs were more than four times greater than actual medical costs; and 2) The true costs of poor health are driven by lifestyle-related factors. The latter were listed as productivity conditions; ten were highlighted:

- Fatigue
- Depression
- Back/neck pain
- Sleeping problem
- Other chronic pain
- Arthritis
- Hypertension
- Obesity
- High cholesterol
- Anxiety

These findings led researchers to urge "health and productivity enhancement strategies." I think this meant teaching REAL wellness skills (e.g., critical thinking, happiness, a deeper understanding of science, meaning and purpose and ethics). The idea: boost individual worker and company performance, along with quality of life for everyone.

From a manager's perspective, medically-based risk reduction seems a safe bet. Who would oppose early detection, disease management and the other preventive-type initiatives designed to encourage the workforce to behave less badly while learning more about health problems? Prevention does some good, costs relatively little and does not stir up waves (i.e., controversies).

But, what about the average person who does not feel a need for classes in weight loss, smoking cessation or other remedial problem areas? How about the employee who finds health hazard appraisals boring if not a time-waster?

What about the physically active employee who practices a sensible lifestyle, engages in no risky behaviors and does not need classes in disease-oriented subjects (as in the ten disorders list given above)? He or she will not find traditional worksite wellness of much use. If the company offers a wellness center with excellent sports facilities, that's an attraction, of course, but the rest of the prevention-dominated corporate wellness menu has little appeal. What can a concerned employee do in such a situation?

Lobby, campaign, plot, connive, demand or otherwise work to encourage your company to move worksite wellness to the next level—to REAL wellness designed for quality of life enhancement. A REAL wellness agenda at the worksite is most likely to improve employee health and productivity.

One can never know too much about REAL wellness quality of life topics. These are prime topics for the examined life. These are talents, really—assets of life that if properly presented would appeal to everyone. I have listed topics of this nature already, but look again at the list.

- Effective decision-making
- The nature of happiness and ways to secure more of it
- Pathways to new and more satisfying experiences
- An exploration of ethics, values and the best ways to evaluate current thinking on morality
- A better appreciation of science, as well as explorations in experiencing a fuller sense of wonder, gratitude and commitment to the common decencies

Addressing such issues requires greater creativity than medical or prevention education. Much of what is included is less subject to black and white outcomes, certainties or resolutions. Some, such as ethical matters, could even lead to heated discussions. These are all arguments *for* introducing such matters and others like them, with skilled facilitators, the better to involve everyone in a REAL wellness agenda that others have shied away from.

Some questions for you:

Do you think it's reasonable for wellness ideas to transcend risk reduction, personal responsibility, exercise and fitness, nutrition, stress and disease management—to include critical thinking, exploration of happiness, joy and pleasure?

Can all this be done in a context of maximum choice or freedoms?

If you think so, don't settle only for these neglected areas—there are countless more, all quite enjoyable. Possibilities include play, sound relationships, emotional intelligence, resilience and understanding how to be a better global citizen. Environmental awareness—however modest the individual role might be in the greater scheme of things—when we all act, our influence can be substantial.

REAL wellness patterns:

Do you think of yourself as a well person? From a wellness perspective, you might nod your head modestly if most of the following statements seem consistent with your situation:

- You have, all things considered (e.g., age, support and plentiful opportunities), a nice body and you're justly proud of your fitness level.

- Your diet is thoughtfully chosen—and high in fruits and vegetables, low in fats and simple sugars.

- Stress is not much of an issue—hardly anything upsets your serenity, at least not for long.

- You have a wonderful sense of humor and most days are filled with fun and play, despite many responsibilities, obligations and duties.

- You love your profession and appreciate your good fortune in having an opportunity to do good work, recognizing that many people struggle to find any work at all in difficult times.

- You are able to express yourself concerning the convictions, principles, goals and other factors that give your life meaning and purpose.

What about normal? Why would you want to be normal? Isn't normal just mediocre or worse, especially in western societies, where roughly two-thirds of the population is overweight or obese? How about middle-age—are you middle-age yet? Before deciding, think about what middle age is—or should be. The consensus among experts is there is no such thing. That's my belief, as well. Nobody can say when middle age (or old age, for that matter) begins, ends or how it would be defined and measured: it's all in your head. Middle age and old age are, in fact, whatever you want them to be or, more likely, whatever you allow them to be.

If you think you are too old to be exceptionally well, or put another way, to be remarkably fit, fun, free and functional, then you will not be very fit, fun, free or able to move about in a highly functional capacity. Expectations reinforce attitudes, behaviors, standards and outcomes. Don't settle for normalcy. Set a higher standard—choose wellness.

Why choose wellness? There are hundreds of reasons but they basically come down to two: the first is that unnecessary, avoidable illness is expensive and dangerous. The costs associated with even moderately, "normal" lifestyles are extraordinary. Thus, avoidance of illness, a negative motivation, is the first reason to choose wellness. A wellness lifestyle will improve your chances of avoiding excess weight (now endured by most Americans) and a long list of related illnesses and diseases.

The positive rationale for choosing wellness is that you will look and feel better, have more energy and a better sex life. Isn't that enough? If not, let me add that you will be fitter, less stressed, have more friends, be a better decision maker, play more often, have more fun and more likely than not thrill at the experience of being alive.

A few more REAL wellness tips:

- Adopt a perspective that embraces responsibility for whatever goes well or poorly. Get on with making the best of things, given conditions that exist. This outlook is much better than succumbing to tendencies to blame, excuse, whine, whimper or shift accountability to someone or something else.

- Do not rely on the health care system for health. Use it wisely to speed recovery from injury or illness. The American and most other so-called "healthcare systems" are not about health at all. Such systems are huge disease and illness-based business largely irrelevant to, if not distractions, from living a wellness lifestyle. No matter how expensive or how wondrous doctors, drugs and the medical system can be when used appropriately, what you do or do not do (in concert with human biology/culture/and your environment) will be the critical variable in affecting your appearance, vitality, exuberance and overall health.

- Go out of your way to experience humor, lightness, fun, joy—good times by whatever name you prefer. Laughter and assorted pleasures strengthen your immune system, metabolize bad vibes and act in a thousand ways to make life richer and fuller.

- Develop a deep and abiding sense of tolerance for diversity of all kinds. This applies to differences in styles, appearances, religions, politics, values and opinions—especially those at variance with your own. This will eliminate the negative stressors that come from attempts to change people to be more like you.

- Find as many people to love as possible. Some of them will probably love you back, or at least be nice to you.

- Do some original thinking about why you are here and what it's all about. Too many accept what they were programmed to think. As a free adult, it's your right to decide for yourself. Make the most of your birthright of freedom of thought, speech and all the rest.

- And lastly, be of service to others—it's good for your health, your happiness and your sense of purpose and satisfaction.

## 4. Nutritional wisdom: a condensed overview

To the extent possible, choose foods that will provide important nutrients and the least hazardous non-nutrients. Even worthy nutrients often come to the store shelf packed with hazardous baggage, including excessive fats, sugars and additives.

For the most part, these non-nutrients in otherwise worthy nutrients are included by manufacturers for their purposes (that is, the manufacturers benefit, such as added shelf life, better appearance). Therefore, these nutrients, excessively burdened with junk should be avoided, which is not so difficult once you learn what to look for, and what to guard against.

Choosing foods that science and conscientious diet experts recommend is a high payoff investment in your good health and satisfaction in looking after yourself and your family. Surely you are aware that the common food patterns that focus on "taste alone—don't fret the consequences" have indisputably been shown to be pernicious to your best future! I don't like to dwell or even address negative matters, but even a REAL wellness promoter sometimes has to do it a little bit—and then hurry back to the positive message.

So, feeling duty-bound, I will tell you that reckless—and hugely popular, fast food patterns are indisputably linked to obesity (I'm sure you've noticed), Type 2 diabetes, heart disease and cancer. The really good news, however, is that it is not too late (for most) to avoid the bad and enjoy the good outcomes if you will go to a bit of effort to make a few changes.

A conscious, informed and energy enhancing diet that makes you look and feel good will boost your ratings in nearly all key health indicators. Yes, preparing healthful meals takes a bit of a commitment, particularly at first, but you will get used to it and wonder why you did not start sooner. Some folks have asked me for tips on getting motivated. There are many possibilities. If you are patriotically oriented (e.g., you like to fly the flag, march in parades, sing the national anthem or cheer for your country during the Olympics), do it for that reason—be a patriot in your own right. After all, it costs a nation a small fortune for government health systems to treat the many millions of citizens who get sick in good measure because they fail to do their part to stay well. Oh, and one other motivating reason to consider healthy diets—you may, despite all the awful things that have been said about what it's like, have a desire to become old someday! I never had such a goal growing up, though I never had a conscious goal not to be old someday, either. It just kind of happened—

sneaked up on me and even though I tried to deny it, it came to pass. Now I want to stay that way—as long as possible.

Being well at any age is great, but staying well when a senior citizen, or a "highly experienced person" or a geezer or whatever you like to call one older than, say, 60, is pretty neat. So many who reach this stage, which is three years more than males born in my day (the 1930's) could expect, are not looking or moving so well. So, being quite healthy now and for an extended (by human standards) future is a good motivator for most people, when they think about it sensibly. And why think otherwise? When you do become old, someday, a sound diet (and high fitness level and a few passions that you can indulge without too much difficulty) will markedly boost the chances that you'll be mobile, feel great and last a long time.

So, take a step or two starting today to improve the quality of your diet, if you need to do so. Be as much of a vegetarian as you can manage—getting needed protein from low fat sources. One comic said he was a vegetarian not because he loved animals, but rather because he hated plants. I love plants, and fruits and grains and nuts and all kinds of foods that are consistent with my need for a high energy fuel system, since I train hard for about an hour every day. There is no way I would want to try to support a triathlon-ready lifestyle on a junk food diet and you probably don't want to try such a thing, either.

Here are a few more little tips that could be useful:

- Any food advertised on TV is probably a good item to avoid. Consider the huge spending on product ads during the World Cup or America's Super Bowl. I remember an ad for a snack *food* called Doritos. Not a single word suggested anything nutritious about this item.

- Another item to avoid is the latest fad diet, especially if accompanied by celebrity endorsements. Glenn Cardwell, an Australian blogger on nutritional science, once stated (in so many words—this is not a quote) that buying a diet best-seller amounts to buying a title, not exhibiting good sense; you are being guided by hope, not the reality of gaining a product that will do more good than harm.

- Be suspicious of all advertised health claims. If a claim about a health benefit tempts you to make a purchase, please take the time to check it out. Doing so is not difficult.

- Adding nutrients to imitation food products is of dubious value. Ever wonder why you don't see vegetables, fruits and whole grains advertised on television? Why do you suppose that is? The profit margins don't permit sellers to do so.

- Try to buy foods at farmers' markets and the periphery of supermarkets. The dangerous stuff is usually in the center aisles, unlike in politics where the hazards are on the Far Left and the Far Right ☺

- Don't be easily fooled. Some healthy foods are rendered semi-toxic by processors. An example is containers of yogurt— which can be loaded with colors, sugar, trans-fats and by-products of nuclear waste. (Just kidding about the last item.)

- Do your own cooking as much as possible. And strive for a variety of foods—set a goal to eat 35 different types of foods a week.

- For snacks, keep nuts, fruit (fresh and dried) and veggies conveniently on hand.

5. **Really neat things to consider that will enhance your quality of life**

   ↓ Resolve to seek more satisfaction from most if not all of the things you do repeatedly, like working and taking care of responsibilities.

- Look into the nature of what science has revealed about the nature of happiness and how to experience more of it. An entire field has grown up around it—it's called "Positive Psychology". It is much more interesting and uplifting that the usual focus of psychology, namely, deviance!

- Consider and better yet, adopt the idea that life can, on frequent occasions, be positively exuberant, even without reliance on alcohol and drugs for this purpose!

- Spend more time exploring life's persistent questions, especially those concerning meaning and purpose. Avoid books, articles and people that are not interesting in how they address this delightful topic. Philosophy should never cause anyone to feel dumb, undereducated or somehow not able to appreciate the questions and issues that matter most.

- Have a look at basic principles of critical thinking that apply in everyday practical ways. There are endless sources. Among my favorites is Carl Sagan's ten-point system for "BS" (Balcony detection kit, found in *The Demon-Haunted World.*)

- Think of a few ways you might help a child, or a few adults, respect the nature of science. Help promote both a better understanding and a higher appreciation for reason and evidence-based decision-making. This wellness skill has profound implications for everyday choices. Examples include whether to spend money on lottery tickets, on unproven medical products or on alternative medical treatments, food supplements and the like.

- Recognize the simple fact that there is randomness in events and circumstances—much of what happens to you and others is not personal, nor is there a "reason" that makes any kind of sense. Things just happen—no grand plan of any kind has to be behind anything. Even now, in the first decade of the 21st century, Stone Age perspectives are still held. Take, for instance, the common expression, "there is a reason for everything." There isn't. Random events occur all the time—nothing personal. Celebrate doubt, skepticism and evidence. As Diderot put it, "incredulity is the beginning of philosophy."

## 6. Value explorations that might boost quality of life

Let me mention a few more ideas that will help you appreciate how profoundly different REAL (**R**eason, **E**xuberance, **A**thleticism, **L**iberty) wellness is from health teachings that focus on treatments, tests and other prevention concerns.

Values can be fun to talk about, explore and fine tune. They are not immutable, set down in childhood forever to be defended from assessment, at all costs. The values we are most likely to honor with practice are those we test and fine-tune, if it seems appropriate to do so.

Let's bring values out in the open, talk about ideas and listen to what others think. Values of most interest might be those dealing with common decencies and ethical standards. A capacity to explore values is a skill, an emotional discipline that promotes reflections about human rights instrumental for democratic societies. The payoff includes more tolerance for differences, mutual understanding and advances in family and community harmony. Examples of common decencies are integrity, trustworthiness, benevolence and fairness.

Integrity includes truthfulness, promise keeping, sincerity and honesty; Trustworthiness includes fidelity, loyalty and dependability. Benevolence involves goodwill, refraining from harming others personally or their property. Fairness encompasses gratitude, accountability, justice, tolerance and cooperation.

Three questions might come to mind at this point: 1) how to get started; 2) how long might it take to become comfortable with value assessments and 3) what are the obstacles?

The answer to each of these questions is, of course, it depends—on a lot of things. Find out and explore the variables, barriers and all the rest. But remember, if it were easy, we'd all be doing it.

## 7. The wonders of perspective for effective thinking

To appreciate perspective as a REAL wellness quality, a little comparison may be helpful.

Compared with the size of Earth, the gas giants in our solar system (Jupiter, Saturn and Uranus) are big, but compared with our Sun, not so big. The Sun? Now that's enormous—but, compared with other stars, not so big. The Sun's diameter is 864,938 miles (1,391,980 km). This is almost 10 times larger than the planet Jupiter and about 109 times as big as the Earth. The volume of the Sun is 1,299,400 times bigger than the volume of the Earth; about 1,300,000 Earths could fit inside the Sun.

As compared to other stars, however, the Sun is about average; red giants like Betelgeuse are about 700 times bigger than our Sun (and roughly 50 times as massive). Betelgeuse is also about 14,000 times brighter than the Sun. Red super giants dwarf the Sun.
Source: Zoom Astronomy
http://www.cointelligence.org/newsletter/comparisons.html

Wellness is a bit like that. Compared with preachy health education and defensive prevention, with diets and fasting and massages and medical tests, wellness ideas are huge. However, in relation to what is possible, what might be, not so big. REAL wellness thinking is *Betelgeuse* to ordinary wellness.

A new perspective for REAL wellness welcomes values, goals, multiple and varied ways of thinking and purposes beyond the ordinary. After all, why settle for pursuits and perspectives short of inspirational and consequential?

## 8. Good health, quality of life and rationality

Among the many elements of positive mental health embraced and promoted within the context of a REAL wellness philosophy are:

- Enthusiasm for independent thinking. Josh Billings (1818-1885) said, "I have lived in this world just long enough to look carefully the second time into things that I am most certain of the first time." Wise words.

- Distrust of superstitions

- Regard for tolerance and pluralism

- Embrace of democratic values and resistance to restrictions on individual rights by organizations, governments or any other entities

- Curiosity and respect for pioneers of human advances

- "The heroes of our history are the scientists and thinkers who explored new horizons and thus improved our understanding of humanity." This statement was put forward in 2008 by The Center for Inquiry Transnational on the occasion of Darwin Day on February 9. The Center expressed the view that Darwin's evolutionary principles "changed forever our perception of the human species and the nature of life."

- In a REAL wellness context, be aware of and participate actively in the assessment and promulgation of ideas such as these. In my view, it's all part of being a healthy person. I suspect you would agree.

## 9. Service to others via outreach—a special opportunity

A proven path to success in sustaining any positive change in habits is to take things at a modest pace. This minimizes stressors and keeps expectations in check, guards against excessive enthusiasms and promotes steady progress. A moderate approach to change is the best guarantee of sustaining success over the long haul.

One additional factor that increases your chances to sustain desired REAL wellness philosophical commitments and physical initiatives for greater fitness is to help others.

A lot of people need help to make changes of a wellness nature. This is true more so than ever in today's climate with the global economic crises, high rates of obesity and chronic disease, and poor conditioning at all age levels.

As a person who understands and appreciates REAL wellness, you are in a position to offer a brighter perspective. Consider playing a modest part—that of promoting a shift in focus. The idea is to redirect attention from assorted problems to wellness opportunities. When the opportunity comes along to offer kindly free advice, seize the day—and tell someone about positive ways forward, not looking back or attempting repairs. The evidence suggests that this shift is more enjoyable and more likely to lead to sustainable change. If you simply model REAL wellness—that is live well and healthfully while enjoying life— everyone will be better off than if limited time and energies are invested in solving old problems.

Here's an example that shows the importance of slow change over time, with a positive goal in mind. The overweight person is more likely to succeed if the end result, the goal, is to achieve something exciting, like finishing a 10K, than trying to lose 30 pounds. But, by training for months or longer with the goal of finishing the race, the loss of weight will occur in the process—as a side effect. The negative factor, in summary, takes care of itself when in the path of a celebratory outcome dearly sought.

A crisis of a personal nature can also spur a reassessment. When things reach a certain point, tolerance for the status quo tends to diminish, and adjustments formerly judged too radical seem more attractive and worth trying.

Your mission of assisting others in promoting quality of life could be as an informal advocate for gradual change over time—in seeking positive outcomes. Most people are mired in lifestyle mediocrity—you can champion the idea that others can, like you, do better and enjoy life more. It's not a hard sell.

Another part of your mission, if you find it appealing, is to advance perspectives on one thing or another based on science, reason and evidence. Help others give expression to their natural curiosities, often gone into hibernation about foundation issues—why we are as we are, how we can better influence our fates while helping ourselves and each other. Adding such matters to the REAL wellness agenda will affect not just better physical health, but greater exuberance in living, improved life satisfactions and better stewardship of the environments.

Finally, challenge orthodoxies, if necessary, that obscure or block paths to joy and happiness. Some may say, "This is not a good time to devote energy to self-improvement and shaping a healthier, happier life. The world is in crisis. I must be serious." Well, that's no good reason. Sure, the planet is in a global recession, unemployment may hit 50 million by year's end, and economies will shrink by two percent and world trade by three percent. Ok, but that leaves 97 percent. People are still buying something; businesses continue to function and everyone still needs stuff.

Cheaper stuff, maybe, but buyers are looking and REAL wellness has plenty to offer at attractive costs.

Also, try to get better at presenting value propositions, articulating why REAL wellness choices are attractive and at making best use of your limited resources (of time, money and changing health status).
An American president (FDR) famously said, "The only thing we have to fear is fear itself." It sounds good but I always considered it a debatable if interesting assertion. Perhaps a little fear of mediocrity might be a healthy fear, particularly if it leads one to better habits.

The steady pursuit of a better, high quality of life can lead to cherished successes.

## 10. Worksite wellness

Companies have encouraged employees to make better lifestyle choices for decades.

The main objectives of wellness programs have been:

1. Identify and reduce behaviors that put employees at higher risks of morbidity and mortality.

2.  Decrease absenteeism, poor performance, turnover and other negative indices that do not add value.

3.  Increase employee effectiveness, job satisfaction, retention and productivity.

Worksite wellness offerings provide employees opportunities to obtain medical testing and health education at work. Examples include smoking cessation, weight loss and a wide range of bad habit amelioration initiatives. All these are good—but not at all REAL wellness in nature. They do not expressly promote quality of life enhancement, rather, they discourage quality of life diminution. Testing is good, testing is important but it does not make anyone healthier. (It does indicate at times the need to do something to avoid getting sicker.)

Programs that lead to fewer behavioral risks are also good, also important, but they do not advance states of well-being, either. Such endeavors prevent or at least discourage health status losses. REAL wellness interventions, education and support initiatives are designed to educate, motivate, inform and inspire employees to adopt and sustain healthful behaviors, not give up bad habits. I'm sure you can appreciate that this is an important distinction.

Is worksite wellness effective?

Evaluations of worksite wellness have measured success by comparing costs in time, labor and funds invested to outcomes associated with these programs. The bottom line for almost all studies is that a pittance has been spent for which modest benefits have been realized. Not earth-shaking but a good result. That is another reason why the time is right to move to the next level—by offering REAL wellness education opportunities.

The quantitative nature of worksite wellness returns has not been determined with high confidence, given the limits of varied assessment studies. One source cites 42 qualified evaluation studies that met ten criteria of worthiness. These reports support a finding of "average reductions in total amount/rates of increase of health plan cost of 25% or more." (Source: Larry Chapman, "Meta-Evaluation of Worksite Health Promotion Economic Return Studies," Art of Health Promotion Newsletter, Vol. 6, No 6, January/February 2003.) Yet, when a group of CEOs met at the World Economic Forum, the consensus was that there was not "any evidence that these programs have had the intended impact on improving health or preventing disease." (Source: CNN Health.com, "Commentary: Getting healthy on the job." April 10, 2009.)

The Wellness Councils of America (WELCOA) is a 20 year-old Omaha-based clearinghouse on worksite wellness. WELCOA reported that 81% of American businesses with 50 or more employees had some form of health promotion program. The most common emphasized exercise, smoking cessation classes, back care programs and stress management. (See "In the Life Expectancy Olympics, America Loses To Japan, France, Australia and 38 Other Countries - But Take Heart - We Spend A Lot More," Seekwellness.com, August 31, 2007.)

What accounts for this enthusiasm, despite limited evidence of effectiveness? I can think of a few explanations:

Medical costs consume at least half of corporate profits. Wellness efforts, even if not really the kind of quality of life efforts emphasized in this book, contain medical costs to some degree. Most firms understand that the challenge is to find a method that enables employees to remain well in the first place.

Much of the illness in the US is directly preventable. WELCOA suggests that 95 percent of spending goes for diagnosis and treatment of illness after it occurs. Isn't it strange that this happens when all agree that at least 70% of illness is preventable?

(The leading causes of death are tobacco use, poor diet and alcohol overuse. I would add lack of sufficient exercise to this list.)

In America, healthcare costs are a big concern for business. No other country spends so lavishly on sickness care—over $2.3 billion dollars—as we do—that's 16 percent of our GDP. Despite such spending, 47 million citizens are unprotected, that is, lack health insurance. Many others are underinsured, vulnerable to catastrophic expenses that can and often do ruin them financially. This situation was dramatized by Michael Moore in a marvelous film entitled, "Sicko."

It should be noted that high illness rates in all parts of the world are often a consequence of dreadful conditions at the worksite that make people sick! Honestly—and I am not referring only to sweatshops set up by huge multinational corporations in third world countries. The workplace in many, if not most, nations contribute to unwellness in many ways. Some are due to employee choices (e.g., long commutes) but most are related to social or other realities (e.g., stressful traffic situations, long business hours, unrealistic management expectations about productivity, pressure to perform heroically and so on). Such conditions leave too little time for quality of life activities that keep people well.

Many employees do not get adequate sleep, a factor that some experts consider one of the most important elements of a wellness lifestyle.

Governments could play a key role. Agencies that are charged with safeguarding public health could take on a new role, that of promoting and assessing REAL wellness programs. Corporate leaders would welcome uniform measures of ROI and health status changes. There could be attractive incentives for demonstrated performance. Perhaps tax credits could be offered, in return for meeting health-enhancing objectives. This could improve the nature of worksite wellness, boost health, save money and produce a greater ROI than seen to date.

It is time to evolve beyond prevention. Employees are ready for more than medical questionnaires, health checks and behavior evaluations focused on medical issues and risk factors. Enough already of preventive care, screenings, education and counseling on disease prevention and management! It is time for more exciting and consequential offerings than appraisals, health fairs, self-help programs, medical newsletters, home fitness products and single topic lectures.

More than medically dominated activities are required to engage workers and their families. People are ready for exciting learning environments that support self-directed excellence and well-being. What's needed now is a shift toward life quality education and support. In varied ways, we can all promote efforts to encourage lifestyle enrichment. Enough on the hazards of this and that—don't you agree the time has come for learning about the dynamics of happiness, humor, play, meaning and purpose, critical thinking, emotional intelligence, self-management and skills for greater success in life? For a change, let's steer clear of medical issues or poor habits (delegate that to the medical departments) in order to focus on qualities needed to live wisely in a complex world.

Making the transition:

How might the workplace be better designed as an environment conducive to REAL wellness promoting positive mental health? Basic factors taken for granted are a good place to start. Start with encouraging everyone to recognize the consequences of long hours, a lengthy commute, sleep deficits, unrealistic productivity expectations, pressures to conform and other such factors. Not everything that blocks the way to increased fulfillment is within the individual's control. There are many transition pathways. To avoid feeling overwhelmed, remember how evolution works—slow changes over time. While change is needed now, progress is helpful, too. A less than dramatic pace may be necessary.

No single approach to REAL wellness is required. Allow employees themselves to brainstorm ways to encourage and support positive lifestyle programming. The menu possibilities for REAL wellness deliberations should be wide-ranging and attractive, regardless of employee circumstances, educational levels and existing health status.

Such a transition can change the tone of workplace life. Imagine worksite discussions about environmental matters, such as climate change. People can come to care deeply about such matters as carbon dioxide emissions and other greenhouse gases, ways to embrace new energy technologies and how to curb energy use—definitely more promising than the tired fare of diets, blood pressure medications and disease data.

A richer worksite agenda—philosophy for everyone!

How about promoting healthier choices not from a health perspective but in the context of learning philosophy? Philosophy does not mean abstract ideas—it can and should be used to introduce everyone to richer possibilities of wise living. We all can think more creatively about what constitutes good, purposeful and happy functioning and perspectives worth pondering regarding pain, grief, failure, loss and death.

Philosophy can stimulate rich dialogues, lead to enriching opinion exchanges and render everything of consequence more interesting.

Experts on classical topics, if given more forums, might be a nice counterweight to media commentators who tend to pander to existing prejudices. Citizens in many countries, especially my own, are poorly served by a simplified bifurcation of liberal/progressive versus conservative views on every issue. Philosophers can help everyone see more shades, perspectives and possibilities. How about introducing fresh commentators with interpretations of events from the minds of Socrates, Democritus, Aristotle, Plato, Epicurus, Protagoras, Lucretius and Epictetus? Of course, no reason to overlook Spinoza, Hobbes, Burke, Erasmus, Hume, Voltaire, Kant, Bentham, Mill, Rousseau, Russell, Dewey, Ingersoll, Paine, Diderot, Clemens (Twain), Eliot, Darwin, Edison, Darrow, Murray, Schweitzer and Einstein, either.

One way to engage more people in discussions of big ideas from great minds is to ask better questions. For the moment, ignore obstacles, barriers and resistance you might expect. How can you create programs that, if attempted, might help employees?

- Make the workday more meaningful and valued
- Create an improved sense of community

- Increase levels of motivation to seek improvements
- Find more passions to nourish
- Become more involved in decisions
- Gain more education, formal and otherwise
- Take more risks and make doing so safe from adverse consequences
- Foster creativity and fun while advancing the company mission
- Render work styles and times more flexible.
- Adapt to change, raise expectations for positive experiences, and reduce stressful ambiguities and uncertainties
- Promote vital skills for personal dynamics (e.g., conflict resolution, consensus building)

You can be a leader in a search for ways to change things leading to better workplace and other environments. We need a culture that values learning not only what is needed to do a job but to enjoy a job—and each other. You can encourage people to look for small changes that might result in a little more happiness, fulfillment and better health.

Jerome Rodale, the founder of the magazine Prevention and the Rodale publishing empire, spent his final moments on earth as a guest on the Dick Cavett Show. According to an account of the episode ("The Day A Guest Died On My Show," St. Petersburg Times, May 13, 2007, p.7.), Rodale had bragged, "I'm in such good health (he was 72) that I fell down a long flight of stairs yesterday and I laughed all the way. I've decided to live to be a hundred. I never felt better in my life!" A few minutes later, he slumped over dead while another guest (New York Post columnist Pete Hamill) was being interviewed.

The moral? I'll go with this: Live every day as fully as you can, and celebrate good health with ample measures of joy and exuberance, in a manner that enhances the chances that you might someday die healthy. Since we all have to die sometime, why not as late in life as possible, at a time when you've never felt better?

## 11. Wellness models past and present

There are many definitions of the word wellness. Every promoter of healthy lifestyles has either created his or her own, or adopted (usually with variations) an established, oft-repeated definition. All are similar, and all are useful as guides to the boundaries and issues addressed in this broad area of lifestyle education.

The situation with regard to wellness models is a bit different. Only a few exist—in part because they take more time to construct and in part, perhaps, because they do not seem as essential to non-theoreticians.

As a result, there are far fewer models of wellness than there are definitions. In fact, the only models to gain much attention over the past 30 years are those that appeared in early wellness books and the one adopted and promoted by the National Wellness Institute (NWI)

The NWI promotes a six-part model, the same construct that was first sketched by NWI president Bill Hettler in 1979.

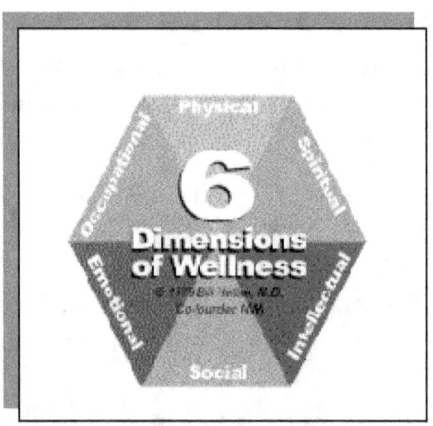

Beginning in 1972, John Travis, MD, developed his Illness-Wellness Continuum to illustrate the relationship of treatment to wellness.

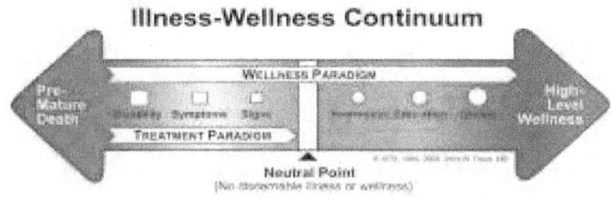

My own model evolved from a simple circle with five dimensions that I introduced in the book, *High Level Wellness: An Alternative to Doctors, Drugs and Disease* (1977, Rodale). It listed the wellness dimensions in a circle, with self-responsibility in the center of that circle, bordered by nutritional awareness, stress management, physical fitness, and environmental sensitivity.

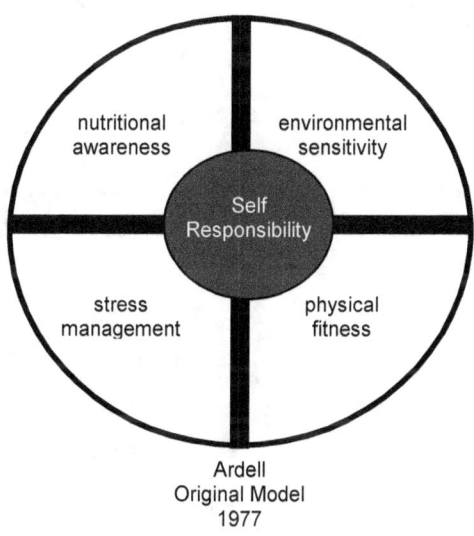

Ardell
Original Model
1977

By 1982, I had decided on a more inclusive classification, which appeared in the book *14 Days to Wellness* (New World Library), as follows: self-responsibility (still in the center), nutritional awareness and physical fitness, meaning and purpose, relationship dynamics, and emotional intelligence.

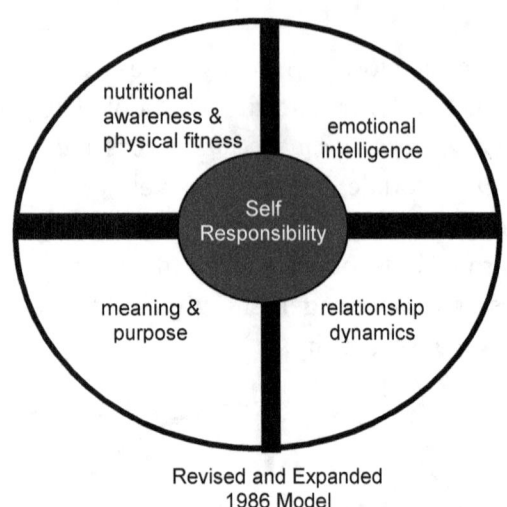

Revised and Expanded
1986 Model

The wellness model below, with 3 domains and 14 skill areas was designed and used from 2000-2009.

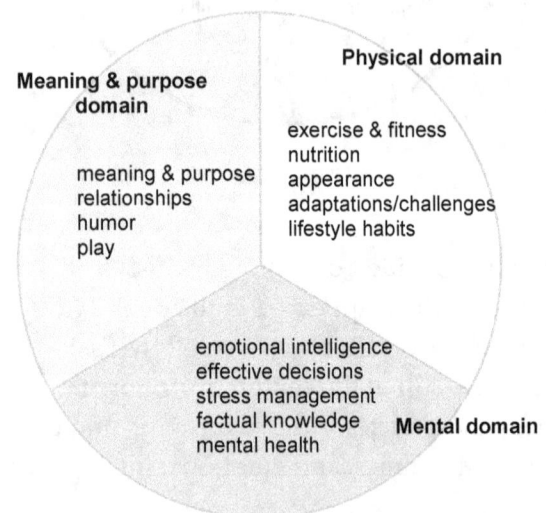

3 Domains & 14 Skill Areas

In 2010, the REAL™ wellness model was developed.

### REAL wellness model

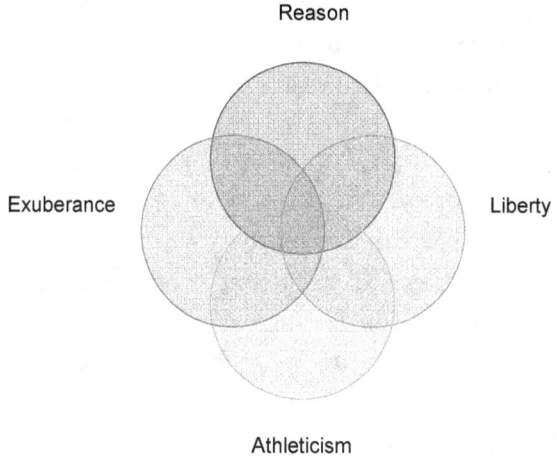

If you feel creative, why not invent your own model of wellness? If you do, send it along to me—I'd love to see and benefit from it. I might even adopt it! Stay open to possibilities—that's the key. What the world needs now are more wellness models, especially if the new models lead to more people leading wellness lifestyles.

## 12. The growth of the wellness movement

The wellness movement got a big boost recently when the spa industry (Global Spa Summit, GSS) released an exciting report. This report describes changes in the way people look after themselves—termed "a paradigm shift from mere reactivity" (i.e., fixing problems) to the pro-activity of wellness. *The Spas and the Global Wellness Market: Synergies and Opportunities,* described the nature and history of wellness, and the way people are beginning to take care of themselves—not only their bodies and minds but their society and their environments. The GSS assessment described the implications and opportunities of these sea changes for the spa industry, projecting a worldwide market worth 1.9 trillion dollars.

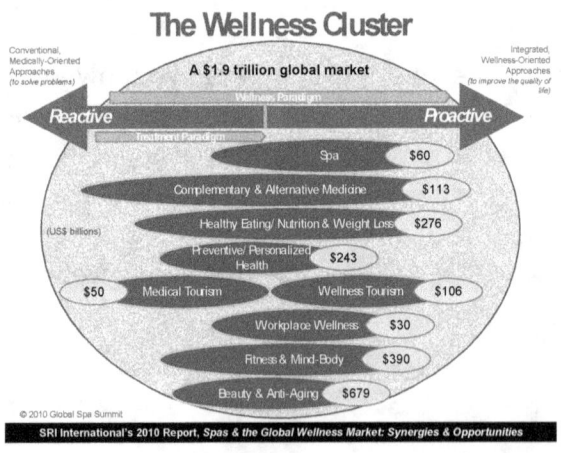

As the wellness movement continues to evolve and grow, I hope this guidebook will be your map to a treasure chest of a healthier and thus better, more enjoyable life.

What is this wellness concept, at its best? I call the advanced variety REAL wellness. Quite simply, REAL wellness is about a terrific lifestyle guided by reason, exuberance, athleticism and liberty. It's designed for living fully, not just preventing illness. It's a lifestyle shaped by effective thinking processes, the purposes of which are happiness and joy within a framework of physical fitness and maximum choices, options and freedoms. An acronym, REAL reflects the key qualities—reason, exuberance, athleticism and liberty. The common alternatives to these states are irrationality, sadness, sedentary functioning and limited choices.

A lifestyle is not a service, remedy or product. It is the way you choose to live. It can't be packaged and sold by a company or vendor. You have to create it. Keep it REAL, that is, rational, fun, active and of your own doing.

Besides reason, exuberance, athleticism and liberty, what do I envision and promote with this guide to an optimal lifestyle?

How about knowledge of and passion for happiness, ethical living, respect for the environment (global awareness) and the thrill of being alive?

This guide has sketched ideas to help you design your own special mindset or philosophy. It has promoted the virtues of using reason as the foundation for decisions, exuberance as the standard for living, athleticism for disciplined daily physical choices and liberty to live your life as you want to live it. It's all about achieving, maintaining and fine-tuning a high quality of life.

REAL wellness is more than non-illness, which is the way most think of health. It's more than an interest in prevention—which basically means a focus on avoiding or reducing the chances of unpleasant situations. REAL wellness is something to work for, to seek—and that is a fulfilling process of living with quality, not seeking a static or unchanging outcome.

The qualities described in the guide set this lifestyle idea apart from the kind of *wellness* that some have tried to associate with taking vitamins, or medical treatments or anything someone else can do to or for you (for a fee, of course).

The point of REAL wellness—the purpose of taking the time and effort to embrace reason, exuberance, athleticism and liberty—is to create and enjoy a better quality of life.

Now you are ready to continue to learn more and varied ways to integrate all kinds of good ideas into decisions for better living.

Parting good wishes:

Real wellness is a philosophy, not a panacea. It promotes reason, exuberance, athleticism and liberty—and it increases our chances to enjoy all the gains and delights that these and other positive qualities entail. Just the same, you will still die someday—and until the end comes you will, regardless of your great attitude, splendid habits, supportive environments and exceptional commitments, have off days. You will even have episodes of illness, suffer bruises physical and emotional and sometimes friends will let you down. But, you knew that. Still, it's a good idea now and then to consciously remember that you are not the center of the universe. It's up to you and a bit of good fortune to remain mostly healthy, happy and out of harm's way. Just do what you can to enjoy each day, investing in your well-being while loving life and special others as much and as long as possible.

Have an epic and triumphant life!

## REAL wellness supplement

The nature of DBRU equivalents

by Donald B. Ardell, Ph.D.

Compared with advances in the medical field, wellness breakthroughs have been slow in coming. Not until about the time of the Renaissance were physicians able to rely on science and not exclusively on healing methods derived from ancient Greek, Chinese, Indian and other systems. When will wellness promoters emerge from the dark ages with comparable leaps forward resulting in epidemics of well-being, veritable plagues of wonderfulness and mass contagions of optimal functioning?

Surely the domains and skill areas associated with wellness and self-management are ripe for new theories, paradigms, constructs and the like. So, where are the Edisons, Fords, Mozarts, Molieres, Einsteins, DaVincis, Franklins, Fermis, Boccaccios, Swifts, Pepys,

Jeffersons, Maughams, Beethovens, Pasteurs and Al Gores (Internet) to lead the way to new visions of wellness?

Well, I'm sure such people will be along shortly. Meanwhile, I have a pretty neat idea.

Of course, wellness breakthroughs, like new theories, paradigms and constructs, are not fashioned anew out of whole cloth, but rather are constructed on the insights and advances of those who came before, to pioneer in modest but vital ways. The art of making art is putting it together, bit by bit and little by little, over time. So, too, it is with pretty neat wellness ideas. Mine was inspired by the creative talent of Gary Larson, the comic genius who gave us the immortal "The Far Side" cartoon series. Specifically, my pretty neat idea, my claim to fame in this life, is based on a Far Side concept that made possible my creation, my invention, my neat idea. I refer, of course, to the concept of the "DBRU equivalent."

The particular "Far Side" cartoon that gave birth to my "DBRU equivalent" was one depicting a large, deceased rhino covered by buzzards with more filling the sky, arriving to join in the feast. In the caption, one buzzard remarks to another, "Just think, here we are, the afternoon sun beating down upon us, a dead bloated rhino underfoot and good friends flying in from all over. I tell you, Frank, this is the best of times."

I looked at that picture, thought of those words and asked myself that question -- that is, what, exactly, ARE "the best of times" in my life? Ever since, I've been asking audiences this question: "Are you getting enough DBRUs? That is, enough dead bloated rhino underfoot equivalents?"

That's my neat idea, my contribution to the advancement of wellness and self-management.

So, what are the best of times for *you*? Put the question to yourself on a regular basis. Ask if you are getting enough DBRU equivalents. What are the best of times in your life and are these experiences occurring with sufficient frequency to make life wonderful? If not, take steps to rectify the situation.

I did one of my famous double-blind, crossover trials of a longitudinal, horizontal and dignified nature a few years ago and discovered we all need a **minimum** daily requirement of 23 DBRU equivalents. They need not be spectacular. Instead, little pleasures, simple reflections of gratitude and conscious appreciations of wonder will do nicely. When you wake, be grateful you are still alive, living in a free country with plenty to eat, that your kids are not in jail (assuming they're not) and that the sun is still up there and that we continue to revolve on planet Earth, not too fast and not too slow. There—you already would have six DBRU equivalents—and you're not even out of bed yet! In other words, DBRU equivalents need not be epic and triumphant events, like recovery from a grave illness, hitting the lottery, winning the Tour De France three times, climbing Mt. Everest in the nude— that sort of thing. Little pleasures throughout the day will do the trick. Tune in to these little delights, bring them into conscious awareness, celebrate them and pause often to honor your good fortune! By the end of the day, you could have pondered hundreds of these wonders, let alone the minimum 23—and you will be richer (and healthier) for it!

I hope this puts you in a good and inquisitive mood for the day and fires up your commitment to take charge of your life and develop a strong interest in self-management. It's time to go out there and celebrate life more than you already do, to seek DBRU equivalents and ways to get fitter, to have more fun and play, richer relationships, more emotional intelligence, to be a more critical thinker and to discover added meanings of and purposes for living, in *your* unique fashion.

As my then high school-age daughter once said to me, "Dad, may all your dead rhinos be like totally bloated on this lovely day."

It's a pity the FDA has not set an RDA standard for DBRU equivalents, but as with other worthwhile initiatives, you don't want to wait for the government to get around to doing the right thing. Seize the day — go out there, identify and enjoy as many DBRU equivalents as possible.

Please consider one more thing. Try to remember that the DBRU concept was not invented, built or written by Thomas Edison, Henry Ford or Wolfgang Amadeus Mozart—or any of those other brilliant folks noted earlier in this essay. No, remember who gave the world the DBRU concept when the time comes to carve another image on Mount Rushmore. Yes, remember who is responsible for the fact that the world knows about and daily enjoys DBRU equivalents—and give Gary Larson his due.